102 Cavity Preventing Juice and Meal Recipes:

Reduce Your Risk of Having Oral Problems Fast and Permanently

By

Joe Correa CSN

COPYRIGHT

This publication is designed to provide accurate and authoritative information in regard to the subject matter covered. It is sold with the understanding that neither the author nor the publisher is engaged in rendering medical advice. If medical advice or assistance is needed, consult with a doctor. This book is considered a guide and should not be used in any way detrimental to your health. Consult with a physician before starting this nutritional plan to make sure it's right for you.

ACKNOWLEDGEMENTS

This book is dedicated to my friends and family that have had mild or serious illnesses so that you may find a solution and make the necessary changes in your life.

102 Cavity Preventing Juice and Meal Recipes:

Reduce Your Risk of Having Oral Problems Fast and Permanently

By

Joe Correa CSN

CONTENTS

ABOUT THE AUTHOR

After years of Research, I honestly believe in the positive effects that proper nutrition can have over the body and mind. My knowledge and experience has helped me live healthier throughout the years and which I have shared with family and friends. The more you know about eating and drinking healthier, the sooner you will want to change your life and eating habits.

Nutrition is a key part in the process of being healthy and living longer so get started today. The first step is the most important and the most significant.

INTRODUCTION

102 Cavity Preventing Juice and Meal Recipes: Reduce Your Risk of Having Oral Problems Fast and Permanently

By Joe Correa CSN

Your teeth and mouth are a reflection of your overall health. What you put in your mouth effects your entire body. Use these oral health revitalizing recipes to start a newer and better life that surprise you in a very positive way.

The first thing that comes to mind when you think about oral health is definitely oral hygiene. Without a doubt, this is the main factor responsible for healthy teeth and the best help you can possibly get in preventing any complications. Brushing daily and flossing keeps your teeth and gums healthy and reduces the chances of having cavities. However, even when we follow our dentist's advice, some complications still happen. The number one culprit for this is usually a bad diet.

Nutrition is the single most important factor affecting your oral health after oral hygiene. The answer lies in having a specific diet full of vitamins, minerals, omega-3 fatty acids, and antioxidants that are proven to build up and strengthen your teeth and that's what this book is all about.

These meal and juice recipes are the solution to your oral problems. Decide to make the change to eat right so that your entire body benefits over time. Your teeth and mouth in general will go over a complete renovative process in a natural and soothing way.

102 CAVITY PREVENTING JUICE AND MEAL RECIPES: REDUCE YOUR RISK OF HAVING ORAL PROBLEMS FAST AND PERMANENTLY

MEALS

1. Warm Basmati Salad

Ingredients:

2 cups of basmati rice

½ cup of spring onions, chopped

¼ cup of fresh cilantro, finely chopped

4 tbsp of apple cider vinegar

2 tbsp of lemon juice, freshly squeezed

¼ tsp of chili pepper, ground

½ tsp of salt

¼ tsp of black pepper, ground

Preparation:

Place the rice in a deep pot. Add about 4 cups of water and bring it to a boil over medium-high temperature. Now, reduce the heat and cover with a lid. Cook for about 40-45 minutes, or until soften.

Meanwhile, combine all other ingredients in a large bowl. Add cooked rice and stir all well to combine. Serve immediately.

Nutrition information per serving: Kcal: 463, Protein: 9.2g, Carbs: 100.4g, Fats: 0.9g

2.   Tomato Beef Stew

Ingredients:

2 lbs of lean beef, cut into bite-sized pieces

2 cups of tomatoes, diced

½ cup of celery, chopped

1 cup of potatoes, peeled and chopped

½ cup of red wine vinegar

2 garlic cloves, finely chopped

1 medium-sized onion

2 tbsp of fresh parsley, finely chopped

3 tbsp of olive oil

½ tsp of salt

¼ tsp of black pepper, ground

Preparation:

Preheat the oil in a large skillet over a medium-high temperature. Add meat and 2-3 tablespoons of water to prevent sticking to the skillet. Cook until slightly browned, and then add onions and garlic. Cook for another minute, then add tomatoes, celery, vinegar, parsley, salt, and pepper. Add water to adjust the thickness. Bring it to a boil then reduce the heat to low. Cook for 40 minutes, then add potatoes. Cook for another 20 minutes. Remove from the heat and serve warm.

Nutrition information per serving: Kcal: 230, Protein: 28.3g, Carbs: 5.3g, Fats: 10.0g

3.   Almond Carrot Smoothie

Ingredients:

1 cup of Greek yogurt

2 medium-sized carrots, sliced

1 medium-sized banana, sliced

2 tbsp of almonds, roughly chopped

Preparation:

Combine carrots, banana, and almonds in a food processor. Blend until for 1 minute, then add yogurt and blend for another minute, or until creamy and smooth. Transfer the mixture to a serving glasses and garnish with some extra almonds. Serve immediately.

Nutrition information per serving: Kcal: 180, Protein: 11.5g, Carbs: 24.4g, Fats: 5.0g

4.   Shrimp Pasta

Ingredients:

1 lb of pasta, whole wheat

2 lbs of shrimps, cleaned and deveined

1 lb of bell peppers, seeded and chopped

3 garlic cloves, crushed

4 tbsp of olive oil

1 large lemon, juiced

1 tsp of lemon zest

½ tsp of sea salt

¼ tsp of black pepper, freshly ground

Preparation:

Preheat the oil in a large nonstick pan over a medium-high temperature. Add garlic and stir-fry for 5 minutes, or until translucent. Now, add shrimps and peppers. Cook for 3-4 minutes then add lemon juice. Sprinkle with some salt and pepper. Cook for a few minutes more, or until heated trough. Remove from the heat and set aside.

Cook pasta using package instructions. Drain well and transfer to a large bowl. Add shrimps and toss to combine. Serve immediately.

Nutrition information per serving: Kcal: 367, Protein: 32.6g, Carbs: 35.0g, Fats: 10.3g

5.   Honey-Herb Turkey

Ingredients:

2 lbs of turkey breasts, thinly sliced

2 garlic cloves, minced

4 tbsp of orange juice

1 tsp of fresh sage, finely chopped

1 tsp of dried thyme, ground

2 tbsp of olive oil

½ cup of honey, raw

¼ tsp of salt

¼ tsp of black pepper, ground

Preparation:

Combine orange juice, sage, thyme, garlic, salt, and pepper in a medium bowl. Stir well and set aside.

Grease a large baking dish with olive oil. Spread the turkey breasts in a dish and pour the half of the honey mixture. Place it in the oven and bake for 30 minutes. Turn over the breasts and add the remaining mixture. Bake for about 25 minutes more. Remove from the heat and serve.

Nutrition information per serving: Kcal: 290, Protein: 26.1g, Carbs: 31.3g, Fats: 7.2g

6.   Cheese Tomato Omelet

Ingredients:

6 large eggs

½ cup of goat's cheese, crumbled

½ cup of cherry tomatoes, diced

1 tbsp of skim milk

3 garlic cloves, minced

1 tbsp of olive oil

½ tsp of salt

¼ tsp of black pepper, ground

Preparation:

Combine eggs, cheese, milk, salt, and pepper in a mixing bowl. Whisk well and set aside.

Preheat the oil in a large frying pan over a medium-high temperature. Add garlic and stir-fry for about 3-4 minutes, or until translucent. Add tomatoes and cook for 2 minutes. Pour the egg mixture and stir once. Cook for 2 minutes, then flip the omelet. Cook for another 2 minutes and remove from the heat. Fold the omelet in half and serve.

Nutrition information per serving: Kcal: 438, Protein: 28.5g, Carbs: 6.0g, Fats: 34.0g

7.   Artichoke Pesto Pasta

Ingredients:

1 cup of artichokes, chopped

1 lb of pasta, pre-cooked

½ cup of Parmesan cheese, grated

2 tbsp of Pecan nuts, roughly chopped

2 garlic cloves, minced

1 cup of fresh basil, chopped

½ cup of parsley, chopped

1 lemon, juiced

4 tbsp of olive oil

½ tsp of kosher salt

¼ tsp of black pepper, ground

Preparation:

Place artichokes in a pot of boiling water. Cook until slightly soften and remove from the heat. Drain well and set aside.

Cook the pasta using package instructions. Drain and transfer to a serving plate.

Meanwhile, combine cheese, nuts, basil, parsley, oil, lemon juice, salt, pepper, and garlic in a food processor. Blend until nice and creamy. Now, add artichokes and re-blend for 1 minute until all well incorporated. Stir in the desired amount of mixture into the pasta and store the rest in a jar and refrigerate.

Nutrition information per serving: Kcal: 586, Protein: 21.8g, Carbs: 69.7g, Fats: 26.1g

8.   Spinach Shitake Mushrooms

Ingredients:

2 cups of fresh spinach, chopped

1 cup of Shitake mushrooms, chopped

1 cup of button mushrooms, chopped

½ cup of cherry tomatoes, chopped

1 cup of Iceberg lettuce, chopped

½ cup of green olives, pitted and halved

2 garlic cloves, minced

4 tbsp of lime juice, freshly squeezed

1 tsp of lime zest

2 tbsp of butter

3 tbsp of extra-virgin olive oil

½ tsp of sea salt

¼ tsp of black pepper, ground

Preparation:

Now, mix together lime juice, vinegar, mustard, oil, salt, and pepper in a mixing bowl. Set aside to allow flavors to mingle.

Melt 1 tablespoon of butter in a medium nonstick saucepan over a medium-high temperature. Add Shitake, button mushrooms and 2 tablespoons of water to prevent sticking to the pan. Cook for 7-10 minutes, or until tender. Transfer the mushrooms to a large salad bowl and reserve the pan.

Melt the remaining butter and add garlic. Stir-fry until translucent. throw in the spinach and cook for 3-4 minutes, or until tender. Remove from the heat and transfer to the bowl with mushrooms.

Now, add tomatoes, lettuce, and olives. Stir once, then drizzle all with previously made dressing. Toss to coat well. Serve immediately.

Nutrition information per serving: Kcal: 252, Protein: 2.8g, Carbs: 12.9g, Fats: 23.2g

9.   Avocado Kale Salad

Ingredients:

1 medium-sized avocado, pitted, peeled and chopped

2 cups of fresh kale, chopped

2 tbsp of lemon juice, freshly squeezed

4 tbsp of orange juice, freshly squeezed

2 tbsp of almonds, roughly chopped

2 tbsp of olive oil

¼ tsp of salt

¼ tsp of black pepper, ground

Preparation:

Combine lemon juice, orange juice, almonds, oil, salt, and pepper in a mixing bowl. Mix well and set aside.

Place kale in a deep pot of boiling water. Sprinkle with some salt and cook for 10 minutes, or until crisp. If you like it more tender, then cook for 20 minutes.

Remove from the heat and drain well. Set aside to cool completely.

Now, combine chopped avocado and kale in a medium salad bowl. Drizzle with the dressing and toss to coat. Garnish with lemon wedges and serve.

Nutrition information per serving: Kcal: 411, Protein: 5.5g, Carbs: 20.6g, Fats: 36.8g

10.   Chicken Basil Pesto

Ingredients:

1 lb of chicken fillets, chopped

1 cup of fresh basil, chopped

4 tbsp of olive oil

¼ cup of tomatoes, sun-dried

2 garlic cloves, minced

3 tbsp of lemon juice, freshly squeezed

¼ tsp of sea salt

¼ tsp of black pepper, ground

Preparation:

Combine all ingredients except olive oil in a food processor and blend for 1 minute, or until nicely incorporated. Gradually add 2 tablespoons of oil and blend again. Set aside.

Preheat the remaining oil in a large nonstick frying pan over a medium-high temperature. add chicken and sprinkle with some salt. Cook for 5 minutes, or until golden brown.

Transfer the chicken to a serving plate and spoon the pesto on top. Serve immediately.

Nutrition information per serving: Kcal: 459, Protein: 44.4g, Carbs: 1.9g, Fats: 30.1g

11.   Beef with Milk Peppers

Ingredients:

1 lbs of beef, cut into bite-sized pieces

½ cup of vegetable broth

2 large bell peppers, chopped

2 tbsp of skim milk

3 garlic cloves, minced

1 large red onion, chopped

2 tbsp of olive oil

1 tsp of Himalayan salt

¼ tsp of black pepper, ground

Preparation:

Preheat the oil in a large nonstick saucepan over a medium high temperature.

Add the meat and cook for 5 minutes, then add vegetable broth. Cook until the liquid evaporates, or until the meat softens. Transfer the meat to a serving plate and reserve the pan.

Add garlic and onion and stir-fry for 3 minutes, or until translucent. Add peppers and sprinkle with salt and pepper to taste. Cook for 3 minutes then add milk. Cook until milk heated trough and remove from the heat. Serve peppers with meat.

Nutrition information per serving: Kcal: 253, Protein: 29.1g, Carbs: 7.5g, Fats: 11.6g

12. Creamy Egg Soup

Ingredients:

3 large eggs

4 cups of chicken broth

1 small carrot, sliced

1 cup of cream cheese

2 tbsp of fresh parsley, finely chopped

1 cup of spring onions, chopped

1 tbsp of cornstarch

¼ tsp of salt

¼ tsp of Cayenne pepper, ground

¼ tsp of salt

Preparation:

Whisk eggs, salt, and pepper in a small bowl and set aside.

Pour the broth into a heavy-bottomed pot. Bring it to a boil and then add cornstarch, carrot, and spring onions. Reduce the heat to low and cover with a lid. Cook for 2 more minutes. Remove from the heat and stir in the cream cheese, parsley, and Cayenne pepper.

Serve warm and reheat the soup if needed.

Nutrition information per serving: Kcal: 181, Protein: 8.3g, Carbs: 4.5g, Fats: 14.5g

13. Broccoli and Cheddar Cheese

Ingredients:

4 cups of broccoli, chopped

1 cup of cheddar cheese, crumbled

1 small onion, finely chopped

4 large eggs

1 cup of skim milk

1 tbsp of olive oil

½ tsp of salt

¼ tsp of black pepper, ground

Preparation:

Preheat the oven to 375°F.

Take a medium baking dish and place some baking paper. Grease with 1 tablespoon of oil and set aside.

Preheat the remaining oil in a large nonstick frying pan over a medium-high temperature. Add broccoli and about 2-3 tablespoons of water to prevent sticking to the pan. Cook for about 7-8 minutes, or until tender. When done, remove from the pan and drain well. Set aside.

Meanwhile, combine eggs, milk, and cheese. Stir well to blend and transfer it to a bowl with broccoli. Give it a good stir and pour the mixture into the baking dish.

Now, take a large baking dish, and pour water in it (about 1 inch will be enough). Place the baking dish in it and place all in the oven. Bake for about 45-50 minutes, or until the toothpick comes out clean after inserted.

Remove from the oven and let it cool for a while. Serve warm.

Nutrition information per serving: Kcal: 221, Protein: 14.5g, Carbs: 9.2g, Fats: 14.5g

14. Kiwi Strawberry Smoothie

Ingredients:

3 large kiwis, peeled and chopped

¼ cup of strawberries, chopped

1 medium-sized banana, chopped

1 cup of Greek yogurt

1 tbsp of honey, raw

Preparation:

Combine all ingredients in a food processor and blend until nicely smooth and creamy. Transfer to a serving glasses and garnish with some nuts or seeds. However, this is optional. Refrigerate for 20 minutes before serving.

Nutrition information per serving: Kcal: 172, Protein: 8.2g, Carbs: 23.0g, Fats: 1.9g

15.   Wild Salmon & Veggie Puree

Ingredients:

2 lbs of wild salmon filets, boneless, thinly sliced

2 cups of sweet potatoes, peeled and chopped

1 small red bell pepper, finely chopped

1 small green pepper, finely chopped

1 tbsp of fresh parsley, finely chopped

4 tbsp of olive oil

2 garlic cloves

1 small red onion, finely chopped

1 tsp of fresh rosemary, finely chopped

1 tsp of sea salt

½ tsp of black pepper, freshly ground

Preparation:

Place potatoes in a pot of boiling water and cook until fork-tender. Remove from the heat and drain well.

Transfer to a food processor and sprinkle with salt. Blend until smooth and place it in a bowl. Add chopped red bell pepper, green bell pepper, red onion, and parsley. Stir all to combine and set aside.

Preheat 2 tablespoons of oil in a large frying pan over a medium-high temperature. Add garlic and stir-fry for 2 minutes and then add meat. Cook for 3 minutes on each side, or until golden crisp. Remove from the heat and set aside.

Mix together the remaining oil, rosemary, salt, and pepper in a small bowl.

Place salmon and potato puree on a serving plate. Drizzle with marinade and serve immediately.

Nutrition information per serving: Kcal: 355, Protein: 30.6g, Carbs: 17.7g, Fats: 18.9g

16.   Ginger Apple Oatmeal

Ingredients:

1 cup of green apples, cut into bite-sized pieces

1 cup of oatmeal

1 cup of skim milk

½ tsp of ginger, ground

1 tbsp of honey, raw

1 tbsp of flaxseeds

Preparation:

Place apples in a pot of boiling water and cook until soft tender. Remove from the heat and drain well. Combine cooked apples, oatmeal, and milk in a deep pot. Cook for 3 minutes, or until heated through. Remove from the heat and stir in the honey. Spoon into serving bowls and top with flaxseeds before serving.

Nutrition information per serving: Kcal: 310, Protein: 10.4g, Carbs: 59.1g, Fats: 4.0g

17.   Turkey Casserole

Ingredients:

1 lb of turkey breasts, skinless and boneless

½ cup of Parmesan cheese, grated

½ cup of chicken broth

1 small carrot, chopped

1 medium-sized tomato, diced

1 tbsp of sour cream

2 tbsp of olive oil

1 tbsp of fresh parsley, finely chopped

1 tbsp of fresh celery, finely chopped

1 tsp of dried thyme, ground

¼ tsp of red pepper flakes

½ tsp of salt

Preparation:

Preheat the oven to 375°F.

Place some baking paper in a casserole dish and sprinkle with some cooking spray.

Preheat the oil in a frying pan over a medium-high temperature. add carrots and cook for 3 minutes, or until slightly tender. Now, add meat and stir in the tomato. Sprinkle with some salt and cook for 5 minutes, then remove from the heat and transfer to a prepared casserole dish. Season with parsley, celery, thyme, salt, and red pepper. Pour the vegetable broth and spread the cheese. Place it in the oven and bake for 20-25 minutes. Remove from the oven and cut into portions. Top with sour cream and serve.

Nutrition information per serving: Kcal: 266, Protein: 26.9g, Carbs: 8.5g, Fats: 14.1g

18.   Pasta Marinara

Ingredients:

2 lbs of pasta

1 large bell pepper, chopped

1 cup of tomatoes, diced

½ cup of tomato paste

1 small onion, finely chopped

2 garlic cloves, minced

1 tbsp of olive oil

1 tbsp of fresh parsley, finely chopped

½ tsp of chili pepper, ground

1 tsp of dried oregano, ground

½ tsp of sea salt

Preparation:

Cook pasta using package instructions. Remove from the heat and drain well. Set aside.

Meanwhile, preheat the oil in a large skillet over a medium-high temperature. Add garlic, onion, and pepper. Sprinkle with some salt to taste. Cook until browned and stir in the tomatoes, parsley, oregano, and chili. Cook for 2 minutes stirring constantly. Now, add tomato sauce and stir until it boils. Remove from the heat and combine with pasta. Toss to coat well and serve.

Nutrition information per serving: Kcal: 492, Protein: 18.8g, Carbs: 91.2g, Fats: 6.1g

19.   Vegetable Tuna Salad

Ingredients:

1 lbs of tuna, minced

1 cup of Iceberg lettuce, chopped

1 small carrot, sliced

1 small onion, finely chopped

¼ cup of cucumber, cubed

1 small red bell pepper, cubed

2 tbsp of extra-virgin olive oil

1 tbsp of fresh parsley, finely chopped

3 tbsp of lemon juice, freshly squeezed

½ tsp of sea salt

¼ tsp of black pepper, ground

Preparation:

Mix together oil, lemon juice, parsley, salt, and pepper in a small bowl. Stir well and set aside to allow flavors to meld.

Meanwhile, combine tuna, carrot, onion, cucumber, and bell pepper in a large bowl. Stir well and drizzle with previously made marinade. Toss all again to coat. Serve immediately.

Nutrition information per serving: Kcal: 299, Protein: 30.9g, Carbs: 6.1g, Fats: 16.4g

20.   Quick Creamy Omelet

Ingredients:

5 large eggs

3 tbsp of sour cream

1 tbsp of fresh parsley, finely chopped

2 tbsp of chives, chopped

1 tbsp of butter

½ tsp of kosher salt

¼ tsp of black pepper, ground

Preparation:

Combine eggs, parsley, chives, salt, and pepper in a medium bowl. Whisk well with a fork and set aside.

Melt the butter in a nonstick frying pan over a medium-low temperature. Pour the egg mixture and cook for 3-5 minutes, stirring constantly. Remove from the heat and stir in the cream. Serve immediately.

Nutrition information per serving: Kcal: 150, Protein: 16.6g, Carbs: 2.1g, Fats: 22.0g

21.   Almond Coconut Cereals

Ingredients:

½ cup of coconut, shredded

1 cup of flaked almonds

1 large banana, sliced

½ cup of almond milk

½ cup of fresh strawberries, chopped

¼ tsp of cinnamon, ground

1 tsp of coconut oil, melted

1 tbsp of liquid honey

Preparation:

Preheat the oven to 300°F.

Combine coconut, almonds, cinnamon, and melted coconut oil.

Spread some parchment paper in a baking dish. Spread the mixture evenly and place it in the oven. Bake for 3 minutes and remove from the oven. Do not overburn. Set aside to cool for a while.

Meanwhile, combine milk, strawberries, banana, and honey in a bowl. Pour this mixture on top of the coconut mixture. Set aside to cool completely and refrigerate for 30 minutes before serving.

Nutrition information per serving: Kcal: 608, Protein: 13.1g, Carbs: 43.7g, Fats: 47.3g

22.   Green Beans Salad

Ingredients:

3 cups of green beans, pre-cooked

3 oz of Feta cheese, crumbled

½ cup of tomatoes, chopped

¼ cup of shallots, chopped

2 tbsp of olive oil

2 tbsp of balsamic vinegar

3 tbsp of fresh basil, chopped

½ tsp of sea salt

¼ tsp of black pepper, ground

Preparation:

Place the beans in a pot of boiling water. Cook until beans tender, then remove from the heat. Drain well and set aside to cool.

Meanwhile, combine oil, vinegar, basil, salt and pepper. Stir well and set aside.

In a large bowl, combine cheese, tomatoes, shallots, and previously cooked beans. Drizzle with dressing and toss to coat. Serve immediately.

Nutrition information per serving: Kcal: 207, Protein: 6.7g, Carbs: 12.7g, Fats: 15.6g

23.   Cranberries Beet Smoothie

Ingredients:

1 cup of fresh cranberries

½ cup of beets, trimmed and pre-cooked

½ cup of spinach, chopped

1 cup of skim milk

1 tsp of fresh mint, chopped

1 tbsp of liquid honey

Preparation:

Place beets in a pot of boiling water and cook until fork-tender. remove from the heat and drain. Set aside to cool completely, or rinse under cold water and drain again.

Now, combine cooked beets, cranberries, spinach, milk, and honey in a food processor. Blend until smooth and transfer to a serving glasses. Garnish with mint and refrigerate for 1 hour before serving.

Nutrition information per serving: Kcal: 128, Protein: 5.0g, Carbs: 24.2g, Fats: 0.1g

24.   Veal Steak with Root Vegetables

Ingredients:

2 lbs of veal steaks

½ cup of celery, chopped

2 large carrots, sliced

½ cup of kohlrabi, trimmed and chopped

¼ cup of fresh parsley, finely chopped

2 tbsp of olive oil

1 tsp of balsamic vinegar

1 tbsp of sour cream

¼ tsp of Cayenne pepper, ground

¼ tsp of black pepper, ground

½ tsp of sea salt

2 tbsp of lemon juice, freshly squeezed

1 tsp of fresh rosemary, finely chopped

Preparation:

Preheat the oven to 425°F.

Combine celery, carrots, kohlrabi, in a pot of boiling water and cook for about 5 minutes, or until tender. Transfer the vegetables to a large baking dish. Drizzle with vinegar, Cayenne pepper, salt and brush with 1 tablespoon of oil. Bake for 3-5 minutes, or until crisp. Remove from the heat and set aside to cool.

Preheat the remaining oil in a large frying pan and add veal steaks. Sprinkle with some salt and cook for 8-10 minutes on both sides, or until golden brown. Remove from the heat and set aside.

Transfer the meat and vegetables to a serving plate. Drizzle with lemon juice and sprinkle with rosemary before serving.

Nutrition information per serving: Kcal: 327, Protein: 40.4g, Carbs: 3.9g, Fats: 15.7g

25. Chicken Zucchini

Ingredients:

1 lb of chicken breasts, skinless and boneless

2 large zucchinis, peeled and chopped

2 garlic cloves, minced

1 small onion, chopped

4 tbsp of olive oil

½ tsp of kosher salt

¼ tsp of black pepper, ground

Preparation:

Place the zucchinis in a pot of boiling water and cook for 2 minutes. Remove from the heat and drain well. Set aside.

Preheat the oil in a large skillet over a medium-high temperature. Add garlic and onion, and stir-fry for about 1 minute. Add meat and cook for 7-10 minutes or until golden brown. Now, add zucchinis and sprinkle with some salt and pepper. Cook for about 2-4 minutes and remove from the heat. Serve chicken with zucchinis.

Nutrition information per serving: Kcal: 247, Protein: 23.4g, Carbs: 5.1g, Fats: 15.1g

26.   Brown Rice with Cheese Sauce

Ingredients:

1 cup of cherry tomatoes, diced

1 cup of brown rice, long-grained

1 cup of Mozzarella cheese, crumbled

1 small onion, chopped

1 tsp of dried oregano, ground

3 tbsp of basil, finely chopped

2 tbsp of balsamic vinegar

2 tbsp of olive oil

½ tsp of salt

¼ tsp of black pepper, ground

Preparation:

Place the rice in a deep pot. Add 2 ½ cups of water and bring it to a boil. Sprinkle with some salt and reduce the heat to low. Cover with a lid and cook for 15 minutes. Remove from the heat and drain the excessive liquid. Set aside to cool completely.

Now, preheat 1 tablespoon of oil in a saucepan over a medium-high temperature. Add onion and stir-fry until translucent. Add tomatoes and cheese and cook until cheese melts. Remove from the heat and stir in the vinegar, oregano, basil, salt, pepper, and remaining oil. Combine rice with this mixture and toss well until incorporated.

Serve immediately.

Nutrition information per serving: Kcal: 361, Protein: 8.4g, Carbs: 53.7g, Fats: 12.9g

27.   Shitake Omelet

Ingredients:

4 large eggs

1 cup of shitake mushrooms, chopped

½ cup of Gouda cheese, roughly grated

1 tbsp of butter

½ tsp of Himalayan pink salt

¼ tsp of black pepper, ground

Preparation:

Whisk the eggs, salt, and pepper in a mixing bowl. Set aside.

Melt the butter in a large frying pan over a medium-high temperature. Add mushrooms and cook for about 8-10 minutes, or until soften. Now, sprinkle with grated cheese and cook for another minute, stirring occasionally. Pour the egg mixture and cook for 3-4 minutes, then flip the omelet. Cook for 2 minutes and remove from the heat. Fold the omelet using a spatula and serve.

Sprinkle with some extra cheese and garnish with fresh parsley.

Nutrition information per serving: Kcal: 412, Protein: 26.3g, Carbs: 12.1g, Fats: 29.6g

28.   Veal Bean Stew

Ingredients:

1 lb of lean veal, cut into bite-sized pieces

1 cup of kidney beans

1 cup of chicken broth

2 small onions, chopped

2 cups of tomatoes, diced

3 tbsp of tomato paste

1 medium-sized bell pepper, diced

2 garlic cloves, crushed

2 tbsp of olive oil

1 tsp of chili pepper, ground

½ tsp of dried thyme, ground

½ tsp of dried oregano, ground

½ tsp of cumin, ground

½ tsp of salt

Preparation:

Preheat the oil in a large nonstick skillet over a medium-high temperature. Add the meat and cook until nicely browned. Now, add onion, garlic and diced bell pepper. Stir and cook for 3 minutes. Add diced tomatoes, and tomato paste. Pour the chicken broth and sprinkle with chili, thyme, oregano, cumin, and salt. Stir all well and cook for about 30-35 minutes. Add water to adjust thickness while cooking. Stir in the beans and cook for 10 more minutes. Remove from the heat and serve warm.

Nutrition information per serving: Kcal: 316, Protein: 27.6g, Carbs: 27.1g, Fats: 11.2g

29.   Grilled Eel

Ingredients:

1 lb of eel, cleaned and cut into bite-sized pieces

4 tbsp of olive oil

2 garlic cloves, crushed

1 small onion, chopped

¼ tsp of Cayenne pepper, ground

4 tbsp of white wine vinegar

1 tbsp of butter

1 tsp of seafood seasoning mix

1 cup of all-purpose flour

1 tsp of fresh rosemary, finely chopped

½ tsp of salt

¼ tsp of black pepper, ground

Preparation:

Combine oil, Cayenne pepper, vinegar, seafood seasoning mix, rosemary, salt, and pepper in a medium bowl. Place the eel chunks in this mixture and toss well to coat. Set aside for 1 hour to allow flavors to penetrate into the meat.

Melt the butter in a large nonstick frying pan over a medium-high temperature. Now, spread the flour on a clean kitchen surface. Spoon the eel on it, draining the marinade. Coat with flour and place it in the frying pan. Fry for 5 minutes, then add onion and garlic. Now, add ½ cup of water and the remaining marinade. Cook for the next 10 minutes, or until the liquid reduced by half.

Remove from the heat and serve immediately.

Nutrition information per serving: Kcal: 541, Protein: 30.4g, Carbs: 26.4g, Fats: 34.2g

30.   Carrot Frittata

Ingredients:

3 large carrots, sliced

6 large eggs

1 cup of spring onions, chopped

2 garlic cloves, minced

½ cup of Gouda cheese, shredded

½ cup of fresh celery, chopped

1 tbsp of olive oil

2 tsp of butter

¼ tsp of dried oregano, ground

½ tsp of kosher salt

¼ tsp of black pepper, ground

Preparation:

Preheat the broiler over a medium-high temperature.

Place the carrots in a pot of boiling water. Add a pinch of salt and cook until tender. Remove from the heat and drain well. Set aside.

Preheat the oil in a large nonstick skillet over a medium-high temperature. Add carrots, spring onions, and garlic. Sprinkle with some salt and pepper and cook for 5 minutes. Remove from the heat and transfer the vegetables to a bowl, but reserve the pan.

Melt the butter in the same skillet over a medium-high temperature.

Meanwhile, mix together eggs, oregano and celery. Season with a pinch of salt and whisk well with a fork. Pour the mixture into the skillet and cook for 3-4 minutes, or until eggs are set. Remove from the heat and top with carrot mixture. Spread the grated cheese and place it under the broiler. Broil for 1 minutes on high until golden brown. Remove and set aside to cool for a while. Serve.

Nutrition information per serving: Kcal: 260, Protein: 15.6g, Carbs: 9.2g, Fats: 18.5g

31.   Raspberry Porridge

Ingredients:

1 cup of rolled oats

1 cup of almond milk

1 cup of water

¼ cup of fresh raspberries

1 large banana, chopped

1 tbsp of sunflower seeds

Preparation:

Pour the water in a medium pot and bring it to a boil. Add oats and cook for 3 minutes, stirring constantly. Remove from the heat and let it soak for 10 minutes.

Now, stir in the almond milk and cook for 1 minute, or until heated trough. Remove from the heat and stir in chopped banana. Top with raspberries and sunflower seeds before serving.

Nutrition information per serving: Kcal: 339, Protein: 6.2g, Carbs: 34.6g, Fats: 21.6g

32.   Beef Burgers

Ingredients:

1 lb of ground beef

1 small onion

¼ tsp of chili pepper, ground

1 tbsp of tomato paste

1 tbsp of fresh parsley, finely chopped

1 tbsp of all-purpose flour

1 garlic clove, minced

¼ tsp of dried oregano, ground

¼ tsp of salt

1 tbsp of sour cream

4 hamburger buns, whole grain

1 tsp of butter

Preparation:

Combine meat, chili, onion, tomato paste, garlic, flour, oregano, salt, and pepper in a large bowl. Mix all with hands and shape the burgers.

Melt the butter in a nonstick skillet over a medium-high temperature. Cook for 6-7 minutes, or until nicely browned. Remove from the heat and set aside.

Place the buns in a toaster and toast for 1 minute. Place the burger on a bottom bun and top with sour cream. Sprinkle with some parsley and cover with a top bun.

Nutrition information per serving: Kcal: 365, Protein: 39.2g, Carbs: 25.7g, Fats: 10.6g

33.   Apple Chia Smoothie

Ingredients:

1 large green apple, cored and chopped

1 cup of skim milk

1 large banana, sliced

¼ tsp of cinnamon

1 tbsp of honey, raw

1 tbsp of chia seeds

Preparation:

Combine all ingredients in a food processor. Blend until creamy and smooth. Transfer to a serving glasses and refrigerate for 30 minutes before serving. Enjoy!

Nutrition information per serving: Kcal: 196, Protein: 5.1g, Carbs: 45.8g, Fats: 0.4g

34.   Cremini Mushroom Polenta

Ingredients:

2 cups of cornstarch

¼ cup of shallots, chopped

2 garlic cloves, crushed

1 lb of cremini mushrooms, thinly sliced

1 tsp of salt

¼ tsp of black pepper, ground

Preparation:

Pour 6 cups of water in a heavy-bottomed pot. Bring it to a boil and gently stir in the cornstarch. Cook for 25 minutes, or until mixture thickens, stirring constantly. Remove from the heat and set aside.

Throw in the onion and shallots in a large nonstick skillet over a medium-high temperature. Cook for 1 minute and then add mushrooms and 3-4 tablespoons of water to prevent sticking to the pan. Sprinkle with salt and pepper and cook for 10 minutes, or until tender.

Serve previously cooked polenta and top with mushrooms. Sprinkle with parsley or top with heavy cream. However, this is optional.

Nutrition information per serving: Kcal: 196, Protein: 5.1g, Carbs: 45.8g, Fats: 0.4g

35.   Stuffed Tomatoes

Ingredients:

4 large tomatoes

¼ cup of leeks, diced

1 cup of brown rice

1 small zucchini, peeled and chopped

3 tbsp of fresh basil, chopped

¼ cup of frozen corn, thawed

2 garlic cloves, minced

4 tbsp of lemon juice, freshly squeezed

½ tsp of salt

¼ tsp of black pepper, ground

Preparation:

Preheat the oven to 350°F.

Place the rice in a deep pot and add 3 cups of water. Bring it to a boil and cook for 15 minutes, or until tender. Remove from the heat and set aside.

Combine leeks, garlic, and 2 tablespoons of water in a large nonstick skillet over a medium-high temperature. Cook for 10 minutes, or until tender. Add zucchini and corn. Stir well and cook for another 2-3 minutes.

Stir in the rice, lemon juice, and basil. Sprinkle with some salt and pepper and cook for 1 minute. Remove from the heat and set aside to cool.

Meanwhile, prepare tomatoes. Cut the top and scoop the flesh. Spoon the mixture to prepared tomatoes. Spread the stuffed tomatoes in a large greased baking dish and bake for about 25-30 minutes.

Nutrition information per serving: Kcal: 228, Protein: 6.2g, Carbs: 47.8g, Fats: 2.0g

36.   Vegetarian Eggplant Steaks

Ingredients:

1 large eggplant, thinly sliced

4 tbsp of lemon juice, freshly squeezed

3 tbsp of balsamic vinegar

3 tbsp of heavy cream

1 cup of arugula, roughly chopped

¼ tsp of black pepper, ground

½ tsp of sea salt

¼ tsp of lemon zest

Preparation:

Preheat the grill to a medium-high temperature.

In a mixing bowl, combine lemon juice, heavy cream, vinegar, and sprinkle with some salt and pepper. Dip the eggplant slices in this marinade and place it on the grill.

Grill for 5 minutes on each side, or until doneness.

Spread the sheet of arugula on a serving plate. Top with grilled eggplants and sprinkle with lemon zest before serving.

Nutrition information per serving: Kcal: 100, Protein: 2.2g, Carbs: 10.3g, Fats: 6.0g

JUICES

1.   Spinach Kiwi Juice

Ingredients:

1 cup of fresh spinach

2 large kiwis, peeled

1 medium-sized apple, cored

1 large cucumber

1 tsp of ginger root

Preparation:

Wash and prepare the ingredients. Run trough a juicer and add few ice cubes before serving.

Enjoy!

Nutrition information per serving: Kcal: 201, Protein: 13.2g, Carbs: 56.5g, Fats: 2.6g

2.   Coco Berry Juice

Ingredients:

1 cup of fresh cranberries

1 cup of fresh strawberries

1 large orange, peeled

2 oz of coconut water

Preparation:

Combine cranberries, strawberries, and orange in a juicer and process until juiced.

Transfer to serving glasses and refrigerate for 30 minutes before serving.

Nutrition information per serving: Kcal: 137, Protein: 3.1g, Carbs: 46.7g, Fats: 0.7g

3.   Carrot Basil Juice

Ingredients:

1 large red apple, cored

2 large carrots

1 cup of fresh basil

1 large red bell pepper, seeded

1 broccoli spear

Preparation:

Wash and prepare all ingredients. Combine all in a juicer and process until juiced.

Transfer to serving glasses and add some ice before serving.

Nutrition information per serving: Kcal: 222, Protein: 8.6g, Carbs: 63.6g, Fats: 1.8g

4.   Pear Apricot Juice

Ingredients:

2 large pears, cored

2 large apricots, pitted

1 large cucumber

1 cup of fresh watercress

1 cup of collard greens

1 large lemon, peeled

Preparation:

Wash and prepare the ingredients. Run trough the juicer, one at a time.

Transfer to serving glasses and add few ice cubes, or refrigerate for 30 minutes before serving. Enjoy!

Nutrition information per serving: Kcal: 293, Protein: 7.1g, Carbs: 96.1g, Fats: 1.7g

5.   Spicy Asparagus Juice

Ingredients:

1 cup of asparagus, trimmed

2 large leeks

1 large artichoke head

1 garlic clove, peeled

1 large cucumber

¼ tsp of Cayenne pepper

¼ tsp of Himalayan salt

Preparation:

Combine asparagus, leeks, artichoke, garlic, and cucumber in a juicer and process until juiced. Transfer to serving glasses and stir in the cayenne pepper and salt.

Serve immediately.

Nutrition information per serving: Kcal: 245, Protein: 14.2g, Carbs: 71.9g, Fats: 1.5g

6.   Leafy Green Juice

Ingredients:

1 cup of celery, chopped

1 cup of mustard greens

1 cup of Romaine lettuce

1 cup of red leaf lettuce

1 cup of butternut squash, cubed

1 cup of Brussel sprouts

1 large lemon, peeled

1 large cucumber

Preparation:

Wash and prepare all ingredients. Run trough the juicer, one at a time.

Transfer to serving glasses and refrigerate for 1 hour before serving.

Enjoy!

Nutrition information per serving: Kcal: 152, Protein: 10.2g, Carbs: 48.4g, Fats: 1.5g

7.   Sweet Berry Juice

Ingredients:

1 cup of fresh blueberries

1 cup of fresh raspberries

1 cup of fresh cranberries

1 large lemon, peeled

1 cup of watermelon, seeded

1 tbsp of liquid honey

Preparation:

Wash and prepare the ingredients. Combine blueberries, raspberries, cranberries, lemon, and watermelon in a juicer and process until juiced.

Transfer to serving glasses and stir in the liquid honey. Add few ice cubes or refrigerate before serving.

Nutrition information per serving: Kcal: 230, Protein: 4.1g, Carbs: 53.1g, Fats: 1.7g

8.   Mango Mint Juice

Ingredients:

1 large mango

1 large cucumber

1 cup of cantaloupe, peeled and cubed

2 tbsp of fresh mint

Preparation:

Combine all ingredients in a juicer and process until juiced. Transfer to serving glasses and add few ice cubes before serving, or refrigerate for 1 hour.

Enjoy!

Nutrition information per serving: Kcal: 268, Protein: 6.1g, Carbs: 74.4g, Fats: 1.9g

9.   Granny Smith's Juice

Ingredients:

1 large Granny Smith apple, cored

1 cup of pineapple chunks

1 cup of cherries, pitted

2 large kiwis, peeled

Preparation:

Wash and prepare the ingredients. Run trough the juicer, one at a time.

Add few ice cubes or refrigerate for 30 minutes before serving.

Nutrition information per serving: Kcal: 287, Protein: 4.2g, Carbs: 84.5g, Fats: 1.2g

10.   Pink Juice

Ingredients:

2 large beets, trimmed

3 large carrots

1 large lemon, peeled

1 medium-sized green apple, cored

3-4 large celery stalks

¼ tsp of ginger, ground

A handful of fresh kale

Preparation:

Combine all ingredients in a juicer and process until juiced. Transfer to serving glasses and stir in the ginger.

Refrigerate for 30 minutes before serving.

Nutrition information per serving: Kcal: 136, Protein: 6.1g, Carbs: 39g, Fats: 1.2g

11.   Avocado Butternut Squash Juice

Ingredients:

1 cup of avocado, peeled, pitted, and cubed

1 cup of butternut squash, cubed

1 cup of fresh basil

1 large orange, peeled

1 large lime, peeled

2 oz of coconut water

Preparation:

Wash and prepare the ingredients. Combine avocado, basil, orange, butternut squash, and lime in a juicer and process until juiced.

Transfer to serving glasses and stir in the coconut water.

Add few ice cubes and serve immediately.

Nutrition information per serving: Kcal: 339, Protein: 6.9g, Carbs: 56.7g, Fats: 21.9g

12.   Grapes and Plums Juice

Ingredients:

2 cups of green grapes

1 cup of fresh plums, pitted

1 large cucumber

1 cup of mustard greens

1 tsp of ginger root

Preparation:

Wash and prepare the ingredients. Combine all in a juicer and process until juiced.

Add few ice cubes or refrigerate before use.

Nutrition information per serving: Kcal: 339, Protein: 6.9g, Carbs: 56.7g, Fats: 21.9g

13. Pumpkin Juice

Ingredients:

1 cup of crookneck squash, cubed

1 cup of pumpkin, cubed

1 cup of butternut squash, cubed

1 large cucumber

1 tsp of ginger, ground

Preparation:

Wash and prepare the ingredients. Combine crookneck squash, pumpkin, butternut squash, and cucumber in a juicer and blend until juiced.

Transfer to serving glasses and stir in the ginger. Refrigerate for 30 minutes, or add few ice cubes and serve immediately.

Nutrition information per serving: Kcal: 140, Protein: 5.8g, Carbs: 40.1g, Fats: 0.9g

14.   Tomato Artichoke Juice

Ingredients:

1 large artichoke head

1 large Roma tomato

1 cup of fresh asparagus, trimmed

1 cup of fresh kale

3 tbsp of fresh parsley, roughly chopped

Preparation:

Wash and prepare the ingredients. Run all trough a juicer, one at a time. Transfer to serving glasses and refrigerate for 30 minutes before serving. garnish with some parsley.

Nutrition information per serving: Kcal: 107, Protein: 13.1g, Carbs: 35.9g, Fats: 1.5g

15.   Pomegranate Watermelon Juice

Ingredients:

1 cup of pomegranate seeds

1 cup of watermelon, seeded

1 cup of beets, trimmed

2 medium-sized radishes

1 medium-sized honeydew melon

1 tbsp of liquid honey

Preparation:

Combine pomegranate seeds, watermelon, beets, radishes, and honeydew melon in a juicer and process until juiced.

Transfer to serving glasses and stir in the liquid honey and add few ice cubes.

Serve immediately.

Nutrition information per serving: Kcal: 167, Protein: 13.1g, Carbs: 45.9g, Fats: 1.5g

16.   Grapefruit Pineapple Juice

Ingredients:

1 large grapefruit, peeled

1 cup of pineapple chunks

1 large cucumber

1 small apple, cored

1 tsp of ginger root

1 large lemon, peeled

Preparation:

Combine all ingredients in a juicer and process until juiced.

Transfer to serving glasses and add few ice cubes or refrigerate for 1 hour before serving.

Nutrition information per serving: Kcal: 280, Protein: 6.1g, Carbs: 84.2g, Fats: 1.3g

17.   Spicy Fennel Kale Juice

Ingredients:

1 fennel bulb, trimmed

1 cup of fresh kale

1 cup of watercress

1 cup of fresh basil

1 large cucumber

3 tbsp of fresh parsley

A handful of spinach

¼ tsp of Cayenne pepper, ground

Preparation:

Wash and prepare all ingredients. Run trough the juicer, one at a time. Transfer to serving glasses and stir in the cayenne pepper.

Refrigerate for 30 minutes before serving.

Nutrition information per serving: Kcal: 280, Protein: 6.1g, Carbs: 84.2g, Fats: 1.3g

18. Beets n' Berries Juice

Ingredients:

1 cup of beets, trimmed

1 cup of blueberries

1 medium-sized apple, cored

2 small carrots

1 large lemon, peeled

2 oz of coconut water

A few mint leaves

Preparation:

Wash and prepare the ingredients. Combine beets, blueberries, apple, carrots, and lemon in a juicer and process until juiced.

Transfer to serving glasses and stir in the coconut water. Garnish with mint and serve.

Nutrition information per serving: Kcal: 240, Protein: 5.6g, Carbs: 74.1g, Fats: 1.5g

19.   Cinnamon Citrus Juice

Ingredients:

3 large orange, peeled

2 large lemons, peeled

2 large limes, peeled

¼ tsp of cinnamon

1 tbsp of liquid honey

2 oz of cold water

Preparation:

Peel the oranges, lemons, and limes. Run trough a juicer and transfer to serving glasses. Add water and stir with a spoon.

Sprinkle with cinnamon and add few ice cubes before serving.

Nutrition information per serving: Kcal: 246, Protein: 6.8g, Carbs: 83.1g, Fats: 1.1g

20.   Cherry Mango Juice

Ingredients:

1 cup of fresh cherries, pitted

1 cup of mango, cubed

1 large lemon, peeled

1 cup of watermelon, cubed

1 tbsp of liquid honey

2 oz of water

Preparation:

Combine cherries, mango, lemon, and watermelon in a juicer and process until juiced.

Transfer to serving glasses and stir in liquid honey and water. Add few ice cubes or refrigerate for 1 hour.

Enjoy!

Nutrition information per serving: Kcal: 288, Protein: 4.6g, Carbs: 68.3g, Fats: 1.3g

21.   Purple Juice

Ingredients:

1 cup of red leaf lettuce

1 large beet, trimmed

1 cup of purple kale

2 large carrots

1 large lemon, peeled

¼ tsp of ginger, ground

Preparation:

Combine all ingredients except ginger and run trough a juicer. Transfer to serving glasses and stir in the ginger.

Refrigerate for 1 hour before serving.

Nutrition information per serving: Kcal: 135, Protein: 7.9g, Carbs: 41.7g, Fats: 1.5g

22.   Swiss Chard Orange Juice

Ingredients:

2 large oranges, peeled

1 cup of Swiss chards

1 large cucumber

4-5 medium celery stalks

1 small lemon, peeled

A handful of parsley

Preparation:

Combine all ingredients in a juicer and process until juiced. Add few ice cubes or refrigerate for 30 minutes before serving.

Nutrition information per serving: Kcal: 214, Protein: 8.4g, Carbs: 67.6g, Fats: 1.5g

23.   Peach and Apricot Juice

Ingredients:

1 large peach, pitted

1 cup of apricots, pitted

1 large cucumber

1 large apple, cored

1-inch piece of ginger root

Preparation:

Wash and prepare all ingredients. Combine all in a juicer and process until juiced.

Add few ice cubes and serve immediately.

Nutrition information per serving: Kcal: 257, Protein: 6.7g, Carbs: 73.3g, Fats: 1.8g

24.   Red Pepper Pineapple Juice

Ingredients:

1 cup of pineapple chunks

2 large carrots

1 large lime, peeled

1 large Granny Smith apple, cored

¼ tsp of red pepper, ground

Preparation:

Combine pineapple, carrots, lime, and apple in a juicer and process until juiced.

Transfer to serving glasses and stir in the red pepper. Add few ice cubes and serve immediately.

Nutrition information per serving: Kcal: 224, Protein: 3.3g, Carbs: 67.1g, Fats: 1.1g

25. Gala Berry Juice

Ingredients:

3 small Gala apples, cored

1 cup of fresh cranberries

1 cup of fresh blueberries

1 cup of fresh kale

1 tbsp of liquid honey

Preparation:

Wash and prepare the ingredients. Combine apples, cranberries, blueberries, and kale in a juicer and process until juiced.

Transfer to serving glasses and stir in the liquid honey. Refrigerate or add few ice cubes before serving.

Nutrition information per serving: Kcal: 368, Protein: 5.6g, Carbs: 106g, Fats: 2.2g

26.   Cherokee Chili Juice

Ingredients:

1 large Cherokee purple tomato

1 cup of beets, trimmed

1 cup of fresh basil

1-inch ginger root

¼ tsp of chili pepper, ground

1 tbsp of fresh parsley, chopped

Preparation:

Combine tomato, beets, basil, and ginger in a juicer and process until juiced.

Transfer to serving glasses and stir in the chili pepper. Garnish with fresh parsley and serve.

You can sprinkle with some salt to taste. However, this is optional.

Nutrition information per serving: Kcal: 99, Protein: 6.4g, Carbs: 28.7g, Fats: 1.2g

27.   Pumpkin Pie Juice

Ingredients:

1 cup of yellow pumpkin, cubed

1 knob of ginger root, (1 inch)

1 medium-sized apple, cored

1 large cucumber

2 large carrots

¼ tsp of cinnamon, ground

Preparation:

Combine pumpkin, ginger, cucumber, and carrots in a juicer and process until juiced. Transfer to serving glasses and refrigerate for 30 minutes before serving.

Enjoy!

Nutrition information per serving: Kcal: 194, Protein: 5.3g, Carbs: 56.1g, Fats: 1.4g

28.   Tropical Juice

Ingredients:

1 ripe avocado, pitted and peeled

1 large guava, peeled

1 large cucumber

1 large lime, peeled

2 oz of coconut water

Preparation:

Combine avocado, guava, cucumber and lime in a juicer and process until juiced. Transfer to serving glasses and stir in the coconut water.

Sprinkle with shredded coconut for decoration. However, this is optional.

Nutrition information per serving: Kcal: 352, Protein: 7.6g, Carbs: 41.6g, Fats: 30.3g

29.   Salted Radish Juice

Ingredients:

5 large radishes, trimmed

1 cup of red leaf lettuce

1 large red bell pepper, seeded

1 large red apple, cored

1 large lemon, peeled

1 cup of watercress

½ tsp of Himalayan salt

Preparation:

Wash and prepare the ingredients. Run trough the juicer, on at a time. Transfer to serving glasses and sprinkle with salt to taste.

Refrigerate before use.

Nutrition information per serving: Kcal: 352, Protein: 7.6g, Carbs: 41.6g, Fats: 30.3g

30. Cilantro Arugula Juice

Ingredients:

½ cup of fresh arugula

½ cup of fresh cilantro

½ cup of fresh spinach

3-4 celery stalks

1 large green apple, cored

Preparation:

Combine all ingredients in a juicer and process until juiced. Transfer to serving glasses.

Refrigerate for 30 minutes before serving.

Nutritional information per serving: Kcal: 61, Protein: 2.1g, Carbs: 20.2g, Fats: 1.2g

31.   Sour Beet Greens Juice

Ingredients:

2 cups of beet greens, trimmed

1 small yellow onion slice

1 cup of fresh celery

3 large leek

1 cup of fresh kale

1 large cucumber

1 ginger knob, (1 inch)

Preparation:

Wash and prepare the ingredients. Combine all in a juicer and process until juiced.

Transfer to a serving glasses and add few ice cubes or refrigerate for 1 hour before serving.

Enjoy!

Nutritional information per serving: Kcal: 230, Protein: 11.5g, Carbs: 63.2g, Fats: 2.1g

32.   Strawberry Mint Juice

Ingredients:

1 cup of fresh strawberries

1 cup of fresh mint

2 medium-sized red apples, cored

1 large honeydew melon wedge

2 oz of coconut water

Preparation:

Combine strawberries, mint, apples and honeydew melon in a juicer and process until juiced.

Transfer to a serving glasses and stir in the coconut water. Add a few ice cubes or refrigerate 1 hour before serving.

Nutritional information per serving: Kcal: 293, Protein: 4.5g, Carbs: 84g, Fats: 1.6g

33.   Cherry Banana Juice

Ingredients:

1 large banana

1 cup of fresh cherries, pitted

2 large red apples, cored

1 cup of watercress

A handful of fresh spinach

Preparation:

Wash and prepare the ingredients. Combine all in a juicer and process until juiced.

Transfer to serving glasses and add few ice cubes. Sprinkle with lemon zest for some extra taste if you like. This is, however, optional.

Enjoy!

Nutritional information per serving: Kcal: 390, Protein: 6.6g, Carbs: 113g, Fats: 1.7g

34.   Tomato Beet Juice

Ingredients:

1 cup of beets, trimmed

2 large tomatoes

1 cup of fresh kale

1 large lemon, peeled

1 rosemary sprig

Preparation:

Combine all ingredients in a juicer and process until juiced.

Transfer to serving glasses and add few ice cubes or refrigerate before serving.

Enjoy!

Nutritional information per serving: Kcal: 125, Protein: 8.9g, Carbs: 38.4g, Fats: 1.7g

35.   Protein Artichoke Juice

Ingredients:

2 large artichokes

1 cup of fresh broccoli

1 cup of mustard greens

1 cup of fresh basil

1 large cucumber

3-4 spinach leaves

¼ tsp of Cayenne pepper, ground

Preparation:

Wash and prepare the vegetables. Run trough a juicer and transfer to serving glasses.

Stir in the Cayenne pepper and serve.

Nutritional information per serving: Kcal: 157, Protein: 18.3g, Carbs: 55.4g, Fats: 1.6g

36.   Black Coconut Juice

Ingredients:

1 cup of fresh blackberries

1 cup of fresh strawberries

1 medium-sized green apple, cored

1 cup of black grapes

2 oz of coconut water

Preparation:

Combine blackberries, strawberries, apple, and grapes in a juicer and blend until juiced.

Transfer to serving glasses and stir in the coconut water. Sprinkle with som shredded coconut for some extra taste, if you like.

Enjoy!

Nutritional information per serving: Kcal: 201, Protein: 4.3g, Carbs: 63.4g, Fats: 1.7g

37.   Spicy Green Juice

Ingredients:

1 cup of fresh broccoli

1 large artichoke head

1 large lime, peeled

1 cup of fresh kale

1 ginger root slice, (1 inch)

¼ tsp of Cayenne pepper, ground

Preparation:

Combine all ingredients in a juicer and process until juiced.

Transfer to serving glasses and stir in the cayenne pepper. Refrigerate for 30 minutes before serving.

Enjoy!

Nutritional information per serving: Kcal: 201, Protein: 4.3g, Carbs: 63.4g, Fats: 1.7g

38.   Parsnip Pepper Juice

Ingredients:

2 cups of parsnips, trimmed

1 large yellow bell pepper, seeded

1 large tomato

1 cup of collard greens

1 large cucumber

Preparation:

Wash and prepare the vegetables. Run trough a juicer and process until juiced.

Transfer to serving glasses and refrigerate for 1 hour before serving.

Enjoy!

Nutritional information per serving: Kcal: 254, Protein: 9.5g, Carbs: 77.7g, Fats: 2.2g

39.   Melon Juice

Ingredients:

1 wedge of honeydew melon

1 cup of watermelon, seeded

1 large cucumber

1 cup of cantaloupe, cubed

1 tbsp of liquid honey

Preparation:

Combine honeydew melon, watermelon, cucumber, and cantaloupe in a juicer and process until juiced.

Transfer to serving glasses and stir in the liquid honey. Add few ice cubes and sprinkle with shredded coconut before serving.

Enjoy!

Nutritional information per serving: Kcal: 201, Protein: 3.4g, Carbs: 57.6g, Fats: 0.8g

40. Carrot Zucchini Juice

Ingredients:

3 large carrots

1 large zucchini, peeled and cubed

1 large orange, peeled

1 cup of pomegranate seeds

1 small ginger root knob, 1 inch

Preparation:

Wash and prepare the ingredients. Run trough the juicer and process until juiced.

Transfer to serving glasses and add some ice before serving.

Enjoy!

Nutritional information per serving: Kcal: 239, Protein: 9.2g, Carbs: 69.7g, Fats: 2.8g

41.   Apple Basil Juice

Ingredients:

2 small golden delicious apples, peeled and seeds removed

1 whole apricot, cored

1 basil leaf

1 cup of collard greens, finely chopped

¼ cup of pure coconut water, unsweetened

Preparation:

Run the ingredients through a juicer and combine with coconut water.

Serve cold.

Nutritional information per serving: Kcal: 144, Protein: 2.3g, Carbs: 44.9g, Fats: 0.9g

42.   Red Raspberry Juice

Ingredients:

2 cups of raspberries

2 cups of red leaf lettuce, shredded

1 cup of watermelon, diced

1 cup of beets, chopped

¼ cup of water

Preparation:

Place the ingredients in a juicer and squeeze. Combine with some water and serve immediately.

Nutritional information per serving: Kcal: 157, Protein: 6.8g, Carbs: 55g, Fats: 2.1g

43.   Pineapple and Grapefruit Juice

Ingredients:

1 cup of pineapple chunks

1 whole grapefruit, peeled

1 large orange, peeled

1 cup of cauliflower, chopped

¼ cup of pure coconut water, unsweetened

Preparation:

Run the ingredients through a juicer.

Add unsweetened coconut water and serve with some ice.

Nutritional information per serving: Kcal: 247, Protein: 6.5g, Carbs: 74g, Fats: 1g

44.   Blueberry and Watercress Juice

Ingredients:

1 cup of watermelon, diced

1 cup of watercress, chopped

1 whole lime, peeled

1 slice of ginger

1 cup of blueberries

Preparation:

Run through a juicer and serve cold.

Nutritional information per serving: Kcal: 129, Protein: 3g, Carbs: 37.4g, Fats: 0.8g

45.　　Sweet Cucumber Juice

Ingredients:

4 large cucumbers, peeled

3 cups of carrots, chopped

2 large oranges, peeled

1 cup of chard, chopped

Preparation:

Place the ingredients in a juicer. Squeeze one at the time and serve immediately.

Nutritional information per serving: Kcal: 283, Protein: 9g, Carbs: 88.9g, Fats: 1.6g

46.   Grapefruit and Cantaloupe Juice

Ingredients:

1 cup of cantaloupe, diced

2 cups of mustard greens, chopped

1 whole grapefruit, peeled

4 cups of parsley, chopped

¼ cup of water

Preparation:

Place the ingredients in a juicer and squeeze.

Add water and serve with some ice.

Enjoy!

Nutritional information per serving: Kcal: 206, Protein: 13.5g, Carbs: 59.3g, Fats: 3g

47.   Mango Juice with Mint

Ingredients:

1 cup of mango, chopped

4 kiwis, peeled

2 cups of kale, chopped

1 tbsp of fresh mint, finely chopped

Preparation:

Run the ingredients through a juicer and serve immediately.

Nutritional information per serving: Kcal: 272, Protein: 10.3g, Carbs: 77g, Fats: 3.3g

48.   Minty Grape Juice

Ingredients:

4 cups of grapes

1 medium-sized zucchini, peeled and chopped

1 cup of watermelon, diced

1 slice of ginger

1 tbsp of fresh mint, finely chopped

Preparation:

Run the ingredients through a juicer and serve cold.

Nutritional information per serving: Kcal: 308, Protein: 5.7g, Carbs: 81.3g, Fats: 2.1g

49.   Crookneck Squash Juice

Ingredients:

4 cups of crookneck squash, sliced

1 large pear, cored

1 cup of green cabbage, shredded

½ cup of pure coconut water, unsweetened

Preparation:

Run through a juicer and combine with unsweetened coconut water.

Serve cold with some ice.

Enjoy.

Nutritional information per serving: Kcal: 192, Protein: 7g, Carbs: 59.9g, Fats: 1.7g

50.   Cherry Juice

Ingredients:

2 cups of cherries, without pits

1 whole grapefruit, peeled

1 whole lime, peeled

1 tbsp of fresh mint, chopped

Preparation:

Wash and prepare the fruits. Run through a juicer and transfer to a serving glass.

Add some ice and serve immediately.

Nutritional information per serving: Kcal: 266, Protein: 5.3g, Carbs: 79.4g, Fats: 1g

51.   Sweet Red Bell Pepper Juice

Ingredients:

2 cups of red bell peppers, chopped and seeds removed

1 cup of blueberries

1 whole lemon

1 large wedge of honeydew melon

Preparation:

Wash the peppers and remove the seeds. Chop them and run through a juicer.

Now add one cup of blueberries, lemon, and honeydew melon.

Run through a juicer and serve cold.

Nutritional information per serving: Kcal: 202, Protein: 5.5g, Carbs: 59.3g, Fats: 1.7g

52.   Green Avocado Juice

Ingredients:

1 cup of avocado, sliced

1 tbsp of fresh mint, finely chopped

1 cup of celery, chopped

1 cup of green cabbage, shredded

½ cup of pure coconut water, unsweetened

Preparation:

Run through a juicer and combine with unsweetened coconut water.

Serve immediately.

Nutritional information per serving: Kcal: 219, Protein: 4.8g, Carbs: 20.8g, Fats: 21.6g

53.   Blueberry Beet Juice

Ingredients:

2 cups of beets

3 cups of beet greens, chopped

1 small banana, peeled

1 cup of blueberries, fresh

Preparation:

Place the ingredients in a juicer, one at the time.

Squeeze and serve immediately.

Nutritional information per serving: Kcal: 242, Protein: 9.1g, Carbs: 75.4g, Fats: 1.4g

54.   Cherry Juice

Ingredients:

2 cups of cherries, without pits

1 whole grapefruit, peeled

1 whole lime, peeled

1 tbsp of fresh mint, chopped

Preparation:

Wash and prepare the fruits. Run through a juicer and transfer to a serving glass.

Add some ice and serve immediately.

Nutritional information per serving: Kcal: 266, Protein: 5.3g, Carbs: 79.4g, Fats: 1g

55.   Sweet Red Bell Pepper Juice

Ingredients:

2 cups of red bell peppers, chopped and seeds removed

1 cup of blueberries

1 whole lemon

1 large wedge of honeydew melon

Preparation:

Wash the peppers and remove the seeds. Chop them and run through a juicer.

Now add one cup of blueberries, lemon, and honeydew melon.

Run through a juicer and serve cold.

Nutritional information per serving: Kcal: 202, Protein: 5.5g, Carbs: 59.3g, Fats: 1.7g

56.   Green Avocado Juice

Ingredients:

1 cup of avocado, sliced

1 tbsp of fresh mint, finely chopped

1 cup of celery, chopped

1 cup of green cabbage, shredded

½ cup of pure coconut water, unsweetened

Preparation:

Run through a juicer and combine with unsweetened coconut water.

Serve immediately.

Nutritional information per serving: Kcal: 219, Protein: 4.8g, Carbs: 20.8g, Fats: 21.6g

57. Plum Tomato Juice

Ingredients:

5 plum tomatoes, halved

1 cup of watercress, torn

1 cup of basil, torn

1 large green bell pepper

1 large cucumber

A handful of spinach

Preparation:

Wash the plum tomatoes and place them in a bowl. Cut in half and reserve the juice while cutting. Set aside.

Combine watercress, basil, and spinach in a colander. Wash thoroughly under cold running water. Drain and torn with hands. Set aside.

Wash the green bell pepper and cut in half. Remove the seeds and chop into small pieces. Set aside.

Wash the cucumber and cut into thick slices. Set aside.

Now, process plum tomatoes, watercress, basil, spinach, green bell pepper, and cucumber in a juicer. Transfer to serving glasses and stir in the salt and water.

Add some ice and serve.

Nutritional information per serving: Kcal: 112, Protein: 8.5g, Carbs: 32.7g, Fats: 1.5g

58. Zucchini Beet Juice

Ingredients:

1 large zucchini

1 cup of beets, trimmed

1 large green apple

1 large radish, trimmed

1 large celery stalk, chopped

2 oz of water

Preparation:

Peel the zucchini and cut in half. Scoop out the seeds and cut into small chunks. Set aside.

Wash the beets and radish. Trim off the green parts and cut into small pieces. Set aside.

Wash the apple and remove the core. Cut into bite-sized pieces and set aside.

Wash the celery and chop it into bite-sized pieces. Set aside.

Now, combine zucchini, beets, apple, radish, and celery in a juicer and process until juiced. Transfer to serving glasses and stir in the water.

Add few ice cubes before serving and enjoy!

Nutritional information per serving: Kcal: 170, Protein: 7.3g, Carbs: 47.9g, Fats: 1.7g

59. Cinnamon Pumpkin Juice

Ingredients:

1 cup of pumpkin chunks

1 large yellow apple, cored

1 large carrot

1 large orange

¼ tsp of cinnamon, ground

3 oz of water

Preparation:

Peel the pumpkin and cut in half. Scoop out the seeds using a spoon. Cut one large wedge and peel it. Cut into small chunks and set aside. Reserve the rest for later.

Wash the carrot and cut into thick slices. Set aside.

Wash the apple and remove the core. Cut into bite-sized pieces and set aside.

Peel the orange and divide into wedges. Set aside.

Now, process pumpkin, apple, carrot, and orange in a juicer. Transfer to serving glasses and stir in the cinnamon and water.

Add few ice cubes and serve immediately.

Enjoy!

Nutritional information per serving: Kcal: 220, Protein: 4.1g, Carbs: 65.3g, Fats: 0.8g

60. Brussels Sprout Crookneck Squash Juice

Ingredients:

1 cup of Brussels sprouts

1 cup of crookneck squash

1 large cucumber

2 large kiwis

1 large lime

3 oz water

1 tbsp of honey

Preparation:

Wash the Brussels sprouts and trim off the outer layers. Cut in half and set aside.

Wash the crookneck squash and cut in half. Scoop out the seeds using a spoon. Cut into small chunks and fill the measuring cup. Reserve the rest for another juice.

Wash the cucumber and cut into thick slices. Set aside.

Peel the kiwis and lime. Cut lengthwise in half and set aside.

Now, combine Brussels sprouts, crookneck squash, cucumber, kiwis, and lime in a juicer and process until juiced.

Transfer to serving glasses and stir in the water and honey. Add some ice or refrigerate for 15 minutes before serving.

Enjoy!

Nutritional information per serving: Kcal: 221, Protein: 7.8g, Carbs: 64.6g, Fats: 1.7g

61.   Ginger Artichoke Juice

Ingredients:

1 large artichoke

1 large grapefruit

1 large honeydew melon wedge

2 large carrots

1 small ginger root knob, 1-inch

2 oz of water

Preparation:

Using a sharp knife, trim off the outer wilted layers of artichoke. Cut into small chunks and set aside.

Peel the grapefruit and divide into wedges. Set aside.

Cut the honeydew melon lengthwise in half. Scoop out the seeds using a spoon. Cut a large wedge and peel it. Cut into small chunks and place in a bowl. Wrap the rest of the melon in a plastic foil and refrigerate.

Wash the carrots and cut into thick slices. Set aside.

Peel the ginger knob and set aside.

Now, process, artichoke, grapefruit, honeydew melon, carrots, and ginger in a juicer.

Transfer to serving glasses and stir in the water. Add some ice and serve immediately.

Nutritional information per serving: Kcal: 230, Protein: 9.5g, Carbs: 72.6g, Fats: 1.1g

62.   Blueberry Strawberry Juice

Ingredients:

1 cup of blueberries

1 cup of strawberries

1 medium-sized green apple, cored

1 large lemon

1 large cucumber

Preparation:

Combine blueberries and strawberries in a colander. Wash under cold running water. Drain and set aside.

Wash the apple and remove the core. Cut into bite-sized pieces and set aside.

Peel the lemon and cut lengthwise in half. Set aside.

Wash the cucumber and cut into thick slices. Set aside.

Now, combine blueberries, strawberries, apple, lemon, and cucumber in a juicer and process until juiced. Transfer to serving glasses and add some ice before serving.

Enjoy!

Nutritional information per serving: Kcal: 284, Protein: 6.8, Carbs: 87.9g, Fats: 2.4g

63.   Avocado Zucchini Juice

Ingredients:

1 cup of avocado, cubed

1 medium-sized zucchini

1 whole leek, chopped

2 medium-sized asparagus spears

3 tbsp of water

Preparation:

Peel the avocado and cut lengthwise in half. Remove the core and cut into small cubes. Fill the measuring cup and reserve the rest in the refrigerator.

Peel the zucchini and cut into bite-sized pieces. Set aside.

Wash the leek and cut into small pieces. Set aside.

Now, combine avocado, zucchini, leek, and asparagus in a juicer and process until juiced. Transfer to a serving glass and stir in the water.

Refrigerate for 10 minutes before serving.

Nutrition information per serving: Kcal: 277, Protein: 22.9g, Carbs: 32.7g, Fats: 22.9g

64.   Pineapple Mint Juice

Ingredients:

1 cup of pineapple, chunked

1 cup of fresh mint, torn

1 cup of watercress, chopped

1 cup of Romaine lettuce, torn

¼ tsp of ginger, ground

Preparation:

Cut the top of the pineapple and peel it using a sharp paring knife. Peel it and cut into small pieces. Set aside.

Combine watercress, mint, and lettuce in a large colander. Wash thoroughly under cold running water and torn into small pieces. Set aside.

Now, combine pineapple, mint, watercress, and lettuce in a juicer. Process until juiced.

Transfer to a serving glass and add some ice before serving.

Enjoy!

Nutrition information per serving: Kcal: 90, Protein: 3.2g, Carbs: 27.3g, Fats: 0.6g

65.   Melon Ginger Juice

Ingredients:

1 cup of watermelon, diced

1 medium-sized wedge of honeydew melon

1 small ginger knob, peeled and chopped

1 medium-sized carrot, sliced

1 small banana, chunked

Preparation:

Cut the top of the watermelon. Cut lengthwise in half and then cut one large wedge. Peel it and cut into small cubes. Remove the seeds and fill the measuring cup. Wrap the rest in a plastic foil and refrigerate for later.

Cut the melon in half. Cut one large wedge and peel the peel it. Cut into small pieces and set aside. Wrap the rest of the melon in a plastic foil and refrigerate for some other juice.

Peel the ginger and cut into small pieces. Set aside.

Wash and peel the carrot. Cut into thin slices and set aside.

Peel the banana and cut into chunks. Set aside.

Now, combine watermelon, honeydew melon, ginger, carrot, and banana in a juicer. Process until juiced.

Transfer to a serving glass and add some crushed ice before serving.

Enjoy!

Nutrition information per serving: Kcal: 188, Protein: 3.4g, Carbs: 52.8g, Fats: 0.9g

66.   Pear Cucumber Juice

Ingredients:

1 medium-sized pear, cored

1 cup of cucumber, sliced

1 cup of kale, torn

1 small green apple, cored

Preparation:

Wash the pear and cut lengthwise in half. Remove the core and cut into bite-sized pieces.

Wash the cucumber and cut into thin slices. Fill the measuring cup and reserve the rest for later. Set aside.

Wash the kale thoroughly under cold running water and slightly drain. Torn with hands and set aside.

Wash the apple and remove the core. Cut into small pieces and set aside.

Now, combine pear, cucumber, kale, and apple in a juicer and process until juiced. Transfer to a serving glass and add some ice before serving.

Nutrition information per serving: Kcal: 177, Protein: 4.4g, Carbs: 54.5g, Fats: 1.2g

ADDITIONAL TITLES FROM THIS AUTHOR

70 Effective Meal Recipes to Prevent and Solve Being Overweight: Burn Fat Fast by Using Proper Dieting and Smart Nutrition

By

Joe Correa CSN

48 Acne Solving Meal Recipes: The Fast and Natural Path to Fixing Your Acne Problems in Less Than 10 Days!

By

Joe Correa CSN

41 Alzheimer's Preventing Meal Recipes: Reduce or Eliminate Your Alzheimer's Condition in 30 Days or Less!

By

Joe Correa CSN

70 Effective Breast Cancer Meal Recipes: Prevent and Fight Breast Cancer with Smart Nutrition and Powerful Foods

By

Joe Correa CSN

www.ingramcontent.com/pod-product-compliance
Lightning Source LLC
Chambersburg PA
CBHW030251030426
42336CB00009B/346